DON'T BE CONFUSED ABOUT ALL THESE VITAMINS

Among so many different kinds of supplements, it is difficult to choose which kind, how often and how much to take or where to store for how long when considering your vitamin needs. Richard Passwater sorts out misleading information from the tried and true and answers such baffling questions as how to estimate what is required for health insurance, protection from a specific health hazard or for therapy for an existing ailment. His description of each vitamin takes the confusion out of names and labels, and the simple, complete tables make it much easier to understand and determine the optimal level of supplementation for your greatest health.

Richard Passwater, Ph.D., with Earl Mindell, is series editor of the Health Guide series. He is one of the most called-upon authorities for information relating to preventive health care. A noted biochemist, he is credited with popularizing the term "supernutrition" largely as a result of having written two bestsellers on the subject—*Supernutrition: Megavitamin Revolution* and *Supernutrition for Healthy Hearts*. His other books include *Easy No-Flab Diet, Cancer and Its Nutritional Therapies, Selenium as Food & Medicine* and *Trace Elements, Hair Analysis and Nutrition* written with Elmer M. Cranton, M.D.

Earl Mindell, R.Ph., Ph.D., combines the expertise and working experience of a pharmacist with extensive knowledge in most of the nutrition areas. His book *Earl Mindell's Vitamin Bible* is now a million-copy bestseller; and his more recent *Vitamin Bible for Your Kids* may very well duplicate his first *Bible*'s publishing history. Dr. Mindell's popular *Quick & Easy Guide to Better Health* is published by Keats Publishing as well as *The Vitamin Robbers*, a Health Guide.

A Beginner's Introduction to
VITAMINS
THE FUNDAMENTAL NECESSITIES FOR
GROWTH AND MAINTENANCE OF LIFE

by Richard A. Passwater, Ph.D.

Keats Publishing, Inc. New Canaan, Connecticut

A Beginner's Introduction to Vitamins is not intended as medical advice. Its intention is solely informational and educational. Please consult a medical or health professional should the need for one be warranted.

Contents

THE BASIC FACTS ABOUT VITAMINS

Vitamins and minerals are the weak links in most people's nutrition. Government surveys repeatedly show that a large portion of our population is not receiving the recommended amounts of important vitamins and minerals. As the official recommendations are, in the view of many people experienced in nutrition, minimal (see Table 1 for comparisons of suggested vitamin intakes)—barely enough for a non-existent "average" person to avoid serious disease symptoms—such deficiencies present a clear health danger. These surveys also do not include the lesser-known minerals and vitamins, some of which are of considerable nutritional importance.

Why, though, *are* vitamins important? How is it that something you can't taste or see in your food is so crucial in determining what nourishment you get from it? The purpose of this Health Guide is to answer those questions and to explain what vitamins are, what they do, how they work, how many there are, how they are measured, how much of each we need, and how we can get the amount best for us in our diet. We will take the confusion out of vitamin names and labels.

Later, we will examine the reasons why most people aren't getting the recommended amounts of vitamins and how to determine the best amounts for you. We will discuss the optimal level for your greatest health. Let's start at the beginning.

The single most important scientific advance ever made may have been the discovery of vitamins. Even though vitamins are only a minor part of the diet, they play a major role in health. The true value of vitamins is just now being realized, even though they were discovered in the early part of this century. The importance of minerals has not yet been fully realized by most people; they will be discussed in another Good Health Guide.

Q: What are vitamins?

A: The classic definition of a vitamin is a compound that the body needs in trace quantities to maintain life but cannot be made by the body, thus must be obtained in the diet as a constituent of food.

However, that old definition needs modification to adapt to today's better understanding of vitamins.

Vitamins are not a single group of chemicals, but a mixed group of chemical compounds having similar functions. Vitamins are not inorganic minerals, but organic constituents of food. "Organic" is used here according to the chemists' definition—not indicating the type of fertilizer or farming employed. To the chemist, "organic" denotes complex compounds based on molecules of carbon, as are many of the compounds of life in organisms.

Vitamins are defined as being needed in trace quantities, with the meaning "trace" being arbitrary and vague. Traditional nutritionists consider this to be anywhere between a microgram and 100 milligrams (.000001 to 0.1 grams), whereas orthomolecular nutritionists extend the range into several grams.

A complication of the old definition is the phrase "constituents of food." This phrase is meant to indicate that vitamins cannot be made in the body and must be obtained outside the body. However, this does not necessarily require that the vitamins be present in ingested food. Certain vitamins are made by our intestinal bacteria from the food we eat, and we, in turn, absorb these vitamins in sufficient quantities to meet all or most of our needs. Thus, our food supply need not contain such a vitamin though our bodies must be provided with it.

A similar exception to this definition is vitamin D, which can be obtained from dietary sources but is mostly produced from its precursor present in the skin by exposure to sunlight.

If we limit the definition to "trace" quantities, we preclude the possibility that once adequate amounts to prevent deficiency diseases such as scurvy or beriberi are consumed, additional amounts have utility. Vitamins C and E, for example, are considered by many to have health functions beyond those of preventing scurvy or fetal resorption.

Except for the aforementioned qualifications, an accepted definition for a vitamin is:

An organic compound, necessary for growth and maintenance of life, which must be provided in the diet.

Q: How do vitamins work?

A: Vitamins generally do not become incorporated into the body's structure, but assist in carrying out the chemical reactions of life. Therefore they are not required in the same quantity as the structural components, such as proteins, carbohydrates and fats.

Many vitamins are used as part of enzyme molecules. Enzymes control the chemical reactions of life. They perform their function over and over again. They are not used up in these vital reactions, but they do eventually wear out and must be replaced.

You may think of enzymes as something like chemical spark plugs. Spark plugs are critical to the production of energy in motors. The energy comes from the explosive burning of gasoline, not from the spark plugs, yet the gasoline would not ignite without the spark plugs.

At least one vitamin, D, is activated in the body as a hormone-like compound.

Some vitamins may not have roles in enzymes or hormonal-like activity, or it could be that such roles haven't been discovered for them yet.

Vitamin E may serve only to protect body compounds against undesirable reactions.

Our understanding of the various roles of vitamins and how they work is far from complete. However, there are certain specific functions that we do know, and these are listed in Table 2.

Q: How many vitamins are there?

A: At this writing, there are fifteen vitamins accepted as such by the Food and Nutrition Board of the National Academy of Sciences. However, there are a number of "accessory factors" currently under study, and some of them may prove to be true vitamins according to the accepted definition discussed earlier. Still other vitamins may be discovered in the future.

Q: Why are the amounts of vitamins listed in so many different ways? What do they mean?

A: Another point of confusion is that the amounts of vitamin present in foods or supplements are sometimes listed in units of weight such as milligrams or in units of activity such as International Units (I.U.) or United States Pharmacopoeia (USP) units.

During the early period of research on a vitamin, its function may be known but its chemical composition may not be. As an example, the first B vitamin discovered was known to prevent beriberi long before the actual compound could be isolated from rice polishings and identified as thiamine.

Before the active compound is isolated, a scientist can only work with crude material separated from whole foods. At each step in the refinement process, measurements of vitamin activity must be made for each fraction separated to determine where the unknown vitamin is. Weighing the fractions would not provide meaningful information, so samples of each fraction are fed to animals to see how much, if any, vitamin activity they show.

The research on each vitamin led to a different "unit" as an expression of dosage, depending on how the researcher defined its effect on an animal. Thus a series of different units was developed as different researchers used different tests.

Eventually international agreement is reached on units of activity which in turn are defined in terms of the weight of the active compound, once it is identified.

As more knowledge is gained and agreement reached, the dosage is stated in units of weight rather than units of activity. Exceptions to this are made when historical usage is so ingrained that change is resisted or when several forms of the vitamin are in wide usage. Vitamin A is a good example of the former and vitamin E of the latter.

Most vitamins are discussed in terms of milligrams, which is one-thousandth of a gram. It takes 28.3 grams to make an ounce; a rough rule to use with food portions is that 100 grams is equivalent to 3.5 ounces.

Vitamins needed only in extremely small amounts, such as vitamin B12, are usually discussed in terms of micrograms. Micrograms are smaller units of weight than milligrams, as it takes one thousand micrograms to make one milligram. It takes one million micrograms to equal one gram.

Vitamins taken in large doses, often called megadoses, are usually discussed in gram units, such as vitamin C, which may be recommended in doses of several grams.

Q: Why take vitamin supplements? Can't we get all we need from a balanced diet?

A: Too many people are not eating balanced diets. Others have special needs due to genetic deficiencies or poor lifestyles. Some people realize that modern food practices are destroying vitamins in their foods.

The nutritional quality of American diets has been deteriorating at an alarming rate. In 1969, the U.S. Public Health Service released figures from a 12,000-person, ten-state study of people from all walks of life. More nutrients were evaluated than in earlier surveys, but still only five vitamins were covered. Vitamins such as B6 or E are rarely considered in governmental surveys.

The government survey went beyond food consumption tables and utilized blood and urine samples. Gross vitamin deficiencies were confirmed by pathological examinations. Nearly half of the American people were found to be below the official daily Recommended Dietary Allowance (RDA) levels of one or more vitamins or minerals. Nineteen percent of those surveyed were deficient in vitamin B2, 15 percent in vitamin C, 13 percent in vitamin A, and 9 percent in vitamin B1. These deficiencies were similarly distributed throughout all socio-economic levels.

The survey showed that approximately 40 percent of the children 1 to 5 years old and 75 percent of females 18 to 44 years old had vitamin A intakes below the RDA.

Approximately half of the children 1 to 5 years old, and 60 percent of the females 18 to 44 years old had vitamin C intakes below the RDA.

The decline of the American diet can be readily demonstrated by comparing the percentage of those receiving the RDA of various vitamins in three different surveys approximately a decade apart.

In 1955, 80 percent received the RDA for vitamin A; in 1965 the percentage slipped to 74; and in 1972 the percentage plummeted to 28.

In 1955, 78 percent received the RDA for vitamin C; in 1965, 73 percent, by 1972, the percentage fell to 48 percent, less than half of the population.

Many of the links involved in the farm-to-prepared meal process, such as premature harvesting, transportation, storage, processing, canning or freezing/thawing and cooking, produce vitamin loss. However, our greatest problem is choosing not to eat balanced diets.

Stress, strenuous exercise, some medications including birth control pills, and poor living habits, such as heavy drinking and smoking, increase the need for several vitamins. Pregnancy and lactation also require extra nourishment.

Q: How long have we known about the importance of vitamins?

A: Before vitamins were isolated and identified, it was known that the prolonged absence of certain foods from the diet produced fatal diseases. In 1747, the British learned that limes, lemons and oranges prevented and cured scurvy during long voyages. In 1884, the Japanese navy, which had previously subsisted on only white rice, added vegetables, meat and fish to its sailors' diets to prevent beriberi.

However, these events were not accepted by physicians as evidence that these fatal diseases were caused by dietary deficiencies until at least 150 years later. The concept of disease being related to diet was difficult to accept.

Even today when the gross deficiency diseases such as scurvy and beriberi are only rarely seen—thanks to our understanding of nutrition and improved distribution of foods—scientists and physicians still debate a possible role of "subclinical" deficiencies in six of the ten most prevalent fatal diseases.

A French scientist, Jean Dumus, predicted in 1871 that food contained nutrients in addition to protein, fat, carbohydrates and "salts." During the severe food shortage in wartime France, attempts to make artificial milk out of the known nutrients produced disastrous results in children.

In 1905, Pekelharing at the University of Utrecht discovered that mice fed milk and egg protein, rich flour (protein and carbohydrate), lard (fat) and salts (inorganic minerals) could survive for only three to four weeks. When he added milk to the mixture, the mice would remain healthy.

Sir Frederick Hopkins of England concluded in 1906 that "no animal can live on a mixture of proteins, carbohydrates and fats, and even when the necessary inorganic material is carefully supplied, the animal still cannot flourish." Hopkins called these nutrients accessory factors. The concept that additional nutrients in food were related to health was still rejected. Most scientists of the time believed that the problem was due solely to the poor taste of such purified mixtures.

Experiments designed to improve the taste of such refined diets by adding sugar, flavors and eventually butter by Dr. Elmer V. McCollum eventually led to the discovery in 1913 that butter contained a factor that improved the survival time of animals on the purified diets.

The word vitamin was not used until 1911, when Casimir Funk proposed changing the name of this group of nutrients from accessory factors to "vitamines." He wanted to emphasize that the nutrients were vital to life and not merely accessory to other nutrients. The "amine" ending was used because Funk believed that the anti-beriberi factor he isolated from rice polishings belonged to the chemical family called amines, and condensed "vital amines" to "vitamines."

In 1915, it was determined that "two" such factors were missing in the purified diets; one factor was fat-soluble and the other was water-soluble. Today we recognize that there are numerous vitamins of both kinds, and we still use the fat-soluble and water-soluble designations for the vitamins because this classification is useful in predicting how often we need to take the vitamin and whether it is likely to be toxic in large quantities.

Q: Why are vitamin names and numbers so confusing?

A: They are indeed! It is not simply a case of having a few vitamins named by letter designation as they were discovered—vitamin A, vitamin B, vitamin C, vitamin D, vitamin E and vitamin K. There are several vitamin Bs—vitamin B1, vitamin B2, vitamin B3, vitamin B5, vitamin B6 and vitamin B12. They all have important differences in function, and must be thought of as distinct vitamins.

There are also two vitamin A's—vitamin A1 and vitamin A2. They have different chemical structures, but have the same body action and function. They should be thought of as the same; thus the term vitamin A is usually used for either and only rarely does one see the terms vitamin A1 or vitamin A2 on labels. (Beta-carotene is made into vitamin A in the body.)

There is only one vitamin C, but several different chemicals possess vitamin C activity. Vitamin C is best known in the form of ascorbic acid, but it is also available in such substances as sodium ascorbate, potassium ascorbate, calcium ascorbate, zinc ascorbate, etc.

Confused? Hang in there and we'll sort it all out in a moment. Let's continue looking at the mishmash of names and numbers.

Vitamin D has two forms, but they are not called vitamin D1 and vitamin D2. Instead, they are called vitamin D2 and vitamin D3. Why not a vitamin D1? It was a mistake arising from faulty early chemical analysis procedures. The two chemical forms of vitamin D may have significant differences, but you only need one and not both.

You've seen all variations, right? Wrong! Let's look at vitamin E. Vitamin E is not just one chemical, but we don't use numbers as in vitamin E1, vitamin E2, etc. Instead, we use Greek letters as prefixes to vitamin E's chemical name, tocopherol. We have alpha-tocopherol, beta-tocopherol, gamma-tocopherol and so on. And just to be sure to confuse you, we add one or two or both of two letters in front of the Greek letter. Thus we have d-alpha tocopherol or l-alpha tocopherol or dl-alpha tocopherol. The naturally-occurring d-alpha is somewhat more active on a weight basis than the synthetic dl, which is, however, more readily and inexpensively available in supplement form. The avid nutrition buff knows the difference and reads the labels closely to make sure he gets what he wants.

To you as a newcomer, all this can be so intimidating that it prevents you from getting interested or improving your nutritional program. But don't let it be discouraging. Right now, just begin with the basics and ask your retailer for advice. You aren't the only one confused.

This guide will explain the basics, and as you read about nutrition in the future, the terminology will become perfectly clear.

Did you notice that vitamin F, vitamin G and vitamin H were not mentioned? They were renamed or reidentified. But vitamin K is still around, although it was not named following a vitamin J.

Now let's see how all this happened, and go back to Casimir Funk and his "vital amines" or "vitamines."

When the fat-soluble nutrient that cured nutritional eye disease was isolated and designated "A," it was found not to possess an amine group. In 1920, scientists agreed to drop the "e" from "vitamine" and use the term "vitamin" followed by a letter designation. At first letters were assigned alphabetically in order of isolation of the vitamin, but soon some were assigned out of order, such as vitamin K, from the Danish word *Koagulation* and vitamin H (now called biotin), from the German word *Haut* (skin).

In 1956 it was discovered that the original water-soluble vitamin B which prevented beriberi was not a single vitamin but a group of them. Numbers were then added to the letter to designate the separate factors as they were isolated—vitamin B1, vitamin B2, etc.

To compound the terminology confusion, numbers were later added to the fat-soluble vitamins to differentiate between closely related chemical compounds having identical or essentially identical biochemical functions.

Whereas vitamin B1 is completely different in function and composition from vitamin B2, vitamins A1 and A2, as previously mentioned, are essentially the same and are interchangeable dietary components.

Today, the trend is away from the confusing alphanumerical designations toward the use of common chemical names, which are specific for the exact compound referred to. Thus it is correct to discuss the functions of vitamin B3 as a group of two compounds, niacin and niacinamide, or as either of the two chemicals as they might be present in a vitamin tablet. While niacin and niacinamide are thought to possess the same vitamin activity, niacin produces a skin flush, whereas niacinamide does not.

Another advantage of using the common chemical name is that it allows one to expand the classical definition of a vitamin which stresses the need of only trace amounts. For example, vitamins C and E are thought to have functions other than preventing scurvy and sterility. Thus the usage of their chemical names, ascorbic acid and tocopherol, remove mental barriers that spring up in people when the term "vitamin" is used.

Q: What is meant by natural vitamins and synthetic vitamins? Is there a meaningful difference?

A: Perhaps the greatest confusion in the minds of the general public interested in taking vitamin supplements is over the issue of natural versus synthetic vitamins. Much misinformation has been injected into this often very emotionally debated question. A major problem is that various compounds may have similar vitamin activity. For example, the compounds pyridoxine, pyridoxal and pyridoxamine all have vitamin B6 activity. A further complication is that some commercial processes produce materials that possess vitamin activity and consist of mixtures of compounds, some of which are found in nature, some of which are produced only in the synthetic preparation. Vitamin E is such an example—the form that appears in nature can be extracted as "natural" vitamin E or manufactured as a mixture of that form plus another form that does not appear in nature.

The issue is clouded by the realization that isolated vitamins have necessarily been extracted from foods by using many chemical refining processes and that some manufactured vitamins may be contaminated with trace materials that some individuals cannot tolerate. And vitamins extracted from natural sources may be "contaminated" with associated factors that may help the vitamins function or be absorbed by the body. It's possible that some trace "contaminants" may actually be undiscovered nutrients.

Consider the advantage of someone taking vitamin B1 isolated from yeast as opposed to pure thiamine in 1920. The vitamin extracted from yeast provided the other B-complex vitamins unknown at that time.

Keep in mind that your first source of vitamins should be naturally whole, unrefined, unfabricated foods. Eating as many different foods of high nutrient density as possible will insure that you obtain ample quantities of all nutrients, even those still unknown to us. Vitamin supplements can then be added to the diet as a backup measure to compensate for nutrient loss of foods in your diet during storage and cooking, to meet your special needs if such needs are above average, or for added protection against environmental pollutants.

Today many people claim to feel better and feel better protected against environmental pollutants when they take more than the Recommended Dietary Allowance of vitamins. These individuals prefer to take high-potency formulations, which by necessity are highly concentrated.

If one wants to take megadoses of vitamin C in a natural

form such as rose hips, many large tablets are necessary to get the same dosage than can be squeezed into the more compact synthetic formulations.

Scientific tests have found no difference between the natural and synthetic vitamins except as discussed in the case of vitamin E, but in my personal thinking, I trust nature more than I trust our present state of knowledge. Next year we could find a nutritional difference between natural and synthetic vitamin E since there are molecular differences. It is my personal choice to take "natural" vitamin supplements, but I can't justify this choice scientifically.

Don't be confused because natural vitamin C is said to be 30 percent more active than synthetic vitamin C. This is due to the presence of trace amounts of the bioflavonoids. The same increased activity is obtained by adding an equivalent amount of bioflavonoids to the synthetic vitamin C or merely by taking a larger quantity of it.

Q: When should I take my vitamins?
A: With meals unless otherwise directed by a physician. Vitamin supplements are food concentrates and should normally be taken with foods to take advantage of food factors that help absorb vitamins.

Q: How often should I take vitamins?
A: The best results are obtained when the total daily dosage is divided into two or three equal parts. A greater percentage of all the vitamins will be obtained by this practice. Also, since the water-soluble vitamins remain in the body for six to eight hours, a more even blood level is maintained by divided doses.

Q: Where should I store my vitamins?
A: Not in the medicine cabinet in the bathroom, but on the table or near where you store your breakfast cereals.

Q: How long can vitamins be stored?
A: This depends on the formulation and whether or not the package has been opened. Some unopened packages keep 90 percent of their contents' potency for up to five years. More frequently, two years is a typical shelf life. I wouldn't keep an opened bottle more than six months.

Q: How much of each vitamin do I need?

A: Table 1 lists the Recommended Dietary Allowance (RDA) for each vitamin. However, your needs as an individual may be much different from the amounts listed there. Dr. Roger Williams of the University of Texas's Clayton Foundation Biochemical Institute has pointed out that we are all different biochemically. This principle has been demonstrated over and over and is called biochemical individuality. As Dr. Williams stated so eloquently, "We as individuals cannot be averaged with other people. Inborn individuality is a highly significant factor in all our lives—as inescapable as the fact that we are human." Dr. Williams points out that the Recommended Dietary Allowances suggested by the Food and Nutrition Board of the National Academy of Sciences for any five vitamins only *exactly* applies to three percent of the population.

Your body is the best test of what level of each nutrient is best for you. At first you may do well to rely on the RDA table, but as you learn more about your own needs and how your body responds to different diets and different levels of vitamin supplementation, you may wish to tailor your diet and supplement program to optimize your health.

A general rule of thumb is that if you take vitamin supplements as "insurance"—although you feel you eat well and don't wish to read a lot about nutrition—then take a vitamin supplement providing approximately one or two times the RDA.

If you feel that you don't eat as well as you should or wish a little "extra" protection, then you may wish supplements providing two to four times the RDA.

If you wish therapeutic levels, then megadoses of ten times the RDA could be considered. Note the therapeutic recommendations given in Table 1. However, you should be knowledgeable about possible side effects of megadoses of vitamins or monitored by a health professional if you plan to use extremely high therapeutic doses for prolonged periods.

Q: Are vitamins safe?

A: Yes. Of course, anything can be abused and you can get too much of anything. Vitamins A and D can be toxic at very high doses. The beginning level of toxicity varies from person to person. Some adults may find side effects from vitamin A after many months of 30,000 I.U., while most people may not experience side effects at 100,000 I.U. daily. The side effects of vitamin A disappear upon discontinuance. Thus, unless prescribed by a physician, vitamin A should be limited to 25,000 I.U. daily. There is little if any advantage for the normally healthy person to take more than 100 to 500 I.U. of vitamin D daily. Thus, unless prescribed by a physician, vitamin D should be limited to 1,000 I.U. or less daily.

Don't be confused by those who claim that there are thousands of poisonings each year due to overdoses of vitamins. A close examination will show you that this statistic represents *no* vitamin poisonings. This misleading information was once abstracted from emergency department reports of accidental consumption by children of pills that later are found to be vitamins and not some medicine. Vitamins that contain iron can be toxic to children, so they are either protected with child-proof lids or the total amount of iron in the entire bottle will be limited so that there will be no danger even if a child consumes the entire contents.

Q: Can vitamins prevent cancer?

A: Vitamins have been shown to prevent cancer in animals, and surveys indicate that this may also be true for humans. At this writing, studies are under way to answer this question definitely.

Q: My friend who has been a nutrition "buff" for many years says not to take iron with my vitamin E, and not to take calcium and magnesium together. Is this good advice?

A: No. Nature puts all the nutrients together in foods. Whole grains contain vitamin E, iron, magnesium and calcium. Multiple vitamin and mineral supplements also contain all four. Vitamin supplements are food concentrates, and like nutrients in food, are best absorbed when all nutrients are together. Many nutrients help in the assimilation of many other nutrients.

It is true that inorganic iron can partially degrade vitamin E under some "test tube" conditions; this is not a problem in the digestive tract. Inorganic iron and vitamin E are separated, transported differently and protected from each other during digestion and assimilation. It is also true that calcium and magnesium compete with each other for absorption, as do many other minerals, but normal absorption is not perfect anyway. As long as you don't imbalance your mineral intake drastically, nature will take care of the situation by absorbing both.

RECOMMENDED DAILY ADULT VITAMIN INTAKES AS PROPOSED BY DIFFERENT GROUPS OR INDIVIDUALS

This table gives recommended daily adult vitamin intakes as proposed by different groups or individuals. The range is staggering, with, for example, the two government RDAs (there is a difference between the two, but it's not important) considering that 60 milligrams of vitamin C is enough, while others go as high as 3000 for daily use.

There's obviously little agreement, though it is worth noting that most people who have had medical or experimental experience with vitamins agree that substantial multiples of the RDA are usually advisable.

My own recommendations are based on several years of experimental work with animals, though a five-year human test by Drs. Linus Pauling and James Enstrom employing levels of vitamin supplementation of the same order demonstrated a one-third to (for nonsmokers) one-half reduction in normal death rates. Drs. Emanuel Cheraskin, Michael Lesser, Lendon Smith and Robert Atkins derive their suggested intakes from their medical practices and from research; it is noteworthy that Dr. Cheraskin took the unusual step of making a large-scale nutritional survey of healthy people, not patients, in arriving at his recommendations. Dr. Harold Rosenberg, an osteopathic physician, also used the experience of his practice for his suggested supplementation program.

Robert J. Benowicz is a biochemist and Hans J. Kugler, Ph.D., has done extensive vitamin experiments with animals. Durk Pearson and Sandy Shaw are researchers and writers on nutrition.

The books these recommendations are drawn from are listed, along with others on the topic of vitamins, in the Bibliography.

TABLE 1
Adult Vitamin Intakes Recommended by Several Sources

VITAMIN	UNITS	OFFICIAL RDA	FDA USRDA	Passwater (Moderate maintenance)	Passwater (Therapeutic)	Atkins (Basic)	Pearson & Shaw (Life Ext.)	Cheraskin
Vitamin A (retinol)	I.U.	5,000	5,000	10,000-15,000	15,000-25,000	10,000	10,000-20,000	10,000-25,000
Vitamin B1 (thiamine)	mg	1.4	1.5	15-50	50-100	100	250-500	10-25
Vitamin B2 (riboflavin)	mg	1.7	1.7	15-50	50-100	75	100-200	10-25
Vitamin B3 (niacin or niacinamide)	mg	18	20	15-50	50-100	150	3,000	75-150
Vitamin B5 (pantothenic acid)	mg	7	10	50-100	100-500	125	1,000-2,000	50-200
Vitamin B6 (pyridoxine)	mg	2.2	2.0	15-50	50-100	200	250-500	10-25
Vitamin B12 (cyanocobalamin)	mcg	3	6	50-100	50-100	750	500	20-100
Folic Acid	mcg	400	400	800	800	3,600	—	75-100
Biotin	mcg	200	300	250-500	250-500	300	—	25-50
Choline	mg	—	—	25-50	50-200	750	1,000-3,000	100-500

Lesser (Supplemental)	Lesser (Therapeutic)	Benowicz	Smith (Moderate)	Smith (Therapeutic)	Rosenberg	Kugler (Moderate)	Kugler (Therapeutic)
10,000	25,000-100,000	5,000-10,000	5,000-10,000	15,000-30,000	20,000-30,000	10,000-15,000	20,000-30,000
10	1,000	50-150	25-50	100	200-300	14	50
10	up to 5,000	50-150	25-50	100	150-300	17	50
50	100-10,000	100-300	25-50	200-500	400-2,000	180	500
250	500-2,000	100-200	25-50	100-500	100-200	70	200
10	100-1,000	50-150	25-50	50-200	100-400	22	60
100	injection	50-150	25-50	100-1,000	25-75	30	100
400	2,000-40,000	500-1,000	400	400-10,000	2,000-5,000	400	800
—	—	50-150	250-500	250-1,000	300-600	500	500
tbl. lecithin	10,000-20,000	—	25-50	—	250-1,000	—	50

TABLE 1 *continued*
Adult Vitamin Intakes Recommended by Several Sources

VITAMIN	UNITS	OFFICIAL RDA	FDA USRDA	Passwater (Moderate maintenance)	Passwater (Therapeutic)	Atkins (Basic)	Pearson & Shaw (Life Ext.)	Cheraskin
Inositol	mg	—	—	25-50	50-100	450	1,000-3,000	100-500
Para-aminobenzoic acid (PABA)	mg	—	—	25-50	50-100	1,200	1,000-2,000	25-50
Vitamin C (ascorbic acid)	mg	60	60	750-1200	1,000-2,000	1,500	3,000-10,000	1,000-2,500
Vitamin D	I.U.	200	400	100-400	400	400	—	1,000-2,500
Vitamin E (tocopherol)	I.U.	10	30	400	400-1,200	200	500-2,000	600-800
Vitamin K	mcg	140	—	—	—	—	—	—

Lesser (Supplemental)	Lesser (Therapeutic)	Benowicz	Smith (Moderate)	Smith (Therapeutic)	Rosenberg	Kugler (Moderate)	Kugler (Therapeutic)
500	3,000	100-200	25-50	1,000	1,000	—	50
—	2,000	50-150	25-50	25-50	200	—	50
1,000-2,000	2,000-30,000	1,000-2,000	100-500	250-5000	1,000-5,000	600	1,000-2,000
400	1,500-2,800	400-600	400-1,000	400-1,500	800	400	400-600
200-600	600-2,000	100-200	200-400	400 +	800-1200	30-100	200-400
—	200-1600	—	—	—	—	—	—

The amounts of vitamins suggested by most of the authorities in Table 1 can rarely be ingested from ordinary dietary sources; hence the recommendations for supplementation. However, supplementation is just that—something added to what should be an already good diet. Nutrients from natural food sources are in the forms and proportions best assimilated by the body, and almost certainly are accompanied by other valuable substances not yet isolated by researchers. This table gives the best food sources of vitamins and summarizes their functions.

TABLE 2
Vitamin Function and Food Sources

Vitamin	Important sources	Some major physiological functions
Vitamin A (retinol)	Liver, carrots, sweet potatoes, greens, butter, margarine.	Assists formation and maintenance of skin and mucous membranes that line body cavities and tracts, such as nasal passages and intestinal tract, thus increasing resistance to infection. Functions in visual processes and forms visual purple thus promoting healthy eye tissue and eye adaptation in dim light.
Thiamine (B1)	Lean pork, nuts, fortified cereal products.	Aids in utilization of energy. Functions as part of a coenzyme to promote the utilization of carbohydrate. Promotes normal appetite. Contributes to normal functioning of nervous system.

Vitamin	Important sources	Some major physiological functions
Riboflavin (B2)	Liver, milk, yogurt, cottage cheese.	Aids in utilization of energy. Functions as part of a coenzyme in the production of energy within body cells. Promotes healthy skin, eyes and clear vision.
Niacin (B3) (or niacinamide)	Liver, meat, poultry, fish, peanuts, fortified cereal products.	Aids in utilization of energy. Functions as part of a coenzyme in fat synthesis, tissue respiration and utilization of carbohydrate. Promotes healthy skin, nerves and digestive tract. Aids digestion and fosters normal appetite.
Pantothenic acid (B5)	Liver, kidney, egg yolk, meat, milk, whole grain cereals, legumes.	Helps regulate the use of carbohydrate, fat and protein for the production of energy.
Pyridoxine (B6)	Beef, liver, pork, ham, soybeans, lima beans, bananas, whole grain cereals.	Assists in red blood cell regeneration. Helps regulate the use of protein, fat and carbohydrate.
Cyanocobalamin (B12)	Only in animal foods—liver, meat, fish, shellfish, milk, milk products, eggs, poultry— vegetarian diets should include milk or a B12 supplement.	Assists in the maintenance of nerve tissues and normal blood formation.

Vitamin	Important sources	Some major physiological functions
Folic Acid (folacin)	Leafy green vegetables, liver, dry legumes, nuts, whole grain cereals, oranges.	Assists in normal blood formation. Helps enzyme and other biochemical systems function.
Biotin	Kidney and liver, milk, eggs, most fresh vegetables.	Helps regulate the use of carbohydrate. Assists body in forming and using fatty acids.
Choline	Liver, yeast, eggs, grains, organ meats.	Needed for cell membrane structure, transport of fat-soluble substances and nerve impulse transmission.
Inositol	Fruits, cereals, yeast, organ meats, lima beans, peas.	Vitamin function in humans not yet identified.
Para-aminobenzoic acid (PABA)	Liver, yeast, rice, greens, milk, eggs.	Vitamin function in humans not yet identified.
Vitamin C (ascorbic acid)	Broccoli, oranges, grapefruit, papaya, mango, strawberries.	Forms cementing substances, such as collagen that hold body cells together, thus strengthening blood vessels, hastening healing of wounds and bones and increasing resistance to infection. Aids utilization of iron.
Vitamin D	Vitamin D milk, fish liver oils, sunshine on skin (not a food).	Helps absorb calcium from the digestive tract and build calcium and phosphorus into bone.

Vitamin	Important sources	Some major physiological functions
Vitamin E	Vegetable oils, leafy green vegetables, whole grain cereals, wheat germ, egg yolk, butter, milkfat.	Protects vitamin A and unsaturated fatty acids from destruction by oxygen. Exact biochemical mechanism by which it functions still unknown.
Vitamin K	Leafy green vegetables, yogurt.	Needed for blood clotting.

VITAMIN DEFICIENCIES AND SIGNS OF EXCESS

Many opponents of vitamin therapy cite the "dangers" of overdosage. The actual overdosage here is of warning. It's possible to take enough vitamin A to have serious adverse effects, but the amounts involved are massive and unlikely to be taken in any recommended supplementary program. An excess of vitamin B3 can cause a temporary flush, alarming if it's unexpected, but not harmful (indeed, perhaps beneficial). More vitamin C than the body can use causes diarrhea; while unpleasant, it's an excellent indicator that you do have enough C. Bowel tolerance is in fact a standard for diagnostic use in establishing an individual's requirement for the vitamin.

These are the known consequences of vitamin excess; those of deficiency are a good deal worse, up to and including death. This table lists the signs of vitamin under- and over-supply.

TABLE 3
Vitamin Deficiency and Excess Signs

Vitamin	Deficiency signs	Excess signs
Vitamin A	Night blindness, dry, rough skin, eye cornea thickening.	Yellowing of skin and eye whites; painful joint swellings; nausea; dry skin; elevated spinal fluid pressure.

Vitamin	Deficiency signs	Excess signs
Vitamin B1 (thiamine)	Fatigue, insomnia, irritability, loss of appetite, muscle tenderness, lassitude, beriberi.	No side effects known from oral usage.
Vitamin B2 (riboflavin)	Mouth irritation, corner of mouth and lip cracking, magenta-colored tongue, dermatitis, eye redness, exaggerated sensitivity to light.	None known.
Vitamin B3 (niacin or niacinamide)	Loss of appetite, nervousness, mental depression, soreness and redness of the tongue, skin pigmentation, ulceration of the gums, diarrhea, pellagra.	Niacin excess can cause a temporary flushing of the skin, which is not known to be harmful and thought to be beneficial.
Vitamin B5 (pantothenic acid)	Headache, fatigue, muscle cramps, lack of coordination.	None known.
Vitamin B6 (pyridoxine)	Loss of appetite, diarrhea, skin and mouth disorders.	None known.
Vitamin B12 (cyanocobalamin)	Anemia, degeneration of the nervous system.	None known.

Vitamin	Deficiency signs	Excess signs
Folic acid	Anemia, intestinal problems.	None known.
Biotin	Anemia, muscular pain, skin disorders.	None known.
Choline	None known.	None known.
Inositol	None known.	None known.
Para-aminobenzoic acid (PABA)	None known.	None known.
Vitamin C (ascorbic acid)	Bleeding and receding gums, unexplained bruises, slow healing, scurvy.	Diarrhea.
Vitamin D	Loss of appetite, cramps, poor bone formation, rickets.	Unusual thirst, urinary urgency, vomiting, diarrhea.
Vitamin E (tocopherol)	Pigmentation, anemia—no specific deficiency disease recognized.	None known.
Vitamin K	Diarrhea, tendency to bleed.	None known, but abnormal clotting time may result.

BIBLIOGRAPHY

Atkins, R.C., M.D. 1981. *Dr. Atkins' Nutritional Breakthrough*. New York: William Morrow & Co., Inc.

Benowicz, R.J. 1979. *Vitamins and You*. New York: Grosset & Dunlap.

Cheraskin, E., M.D., W. Ringsdorf, D.M.D. and A. Brecher. 1974. *Psychodietetics*. New York: Stein & Day, Publishers.

Clark, L., Revised edition, 1981. *Know Your Nutrition*. New Canaan, CT.: Keats Publishing, Inc.

Food and Drug Administration, Department of Health and Human Services. 1978. *United States Recommended Dietary Allowances*. Washington: The Federal Register.

Food and Nutrition Board, National Research Council. 1980. *Recommended Dietary Allowances: Ninth Revised Edition*. Washington: National Academy of Sciences.

Hoffer, A. and Walker, M. 1980. *Nutrients to Age without Senility*. New Canaan, CT.: Keats Publishing, Inc.

Kugler, H.J., Ph.D. 1978. *Dr. Kugler's Keys to a Longer Life*. New York: Stein & Day, Publishers.

Lesser, M., M.D. 1980. *Nutrition and Vitamin Therapy*. New York: Grove Press, Inc.

Passwater, R., Ph.D. 1975. *Supernutrition: The Megavitamin Revolution*. New York: The Dial Press.

Pearson, D. and S. Shaw. 1982. *Life Extension: A Practical Scientific Approach*. New York: Warner Books, Inc.

Rosenberg, H., D.O., and A.N. Feldzamen, Ph.D. 1974. *The Doctor's Book of Vitamin Therapy*. New York: G.P. Putnam's Sons.

Smith, L., M.D. 1979. *Feed Your Kids Right*. New York: McGraw-Hill, Inc.

Passwater, R., Ph.D. Revised edition, 1983. *Cancer and Its Nutritional Therapies*. New Canaan, CT: Keats Publishing, Inc.

Staff of *Prevention* magazine. 1977. *The Complete Book of Vitamins*. Emmaus, PA: Rodale Press, Inc.

Wade, C. Revised edition. 1983. *Vitamins, Minerals and Other Supplements*. New Canaan, CT: Keats Publishing, Inc.